Basic Bread Machine Cookbook

50 delicious and affordable recipes for your basic bread machine

Raul Wyatt

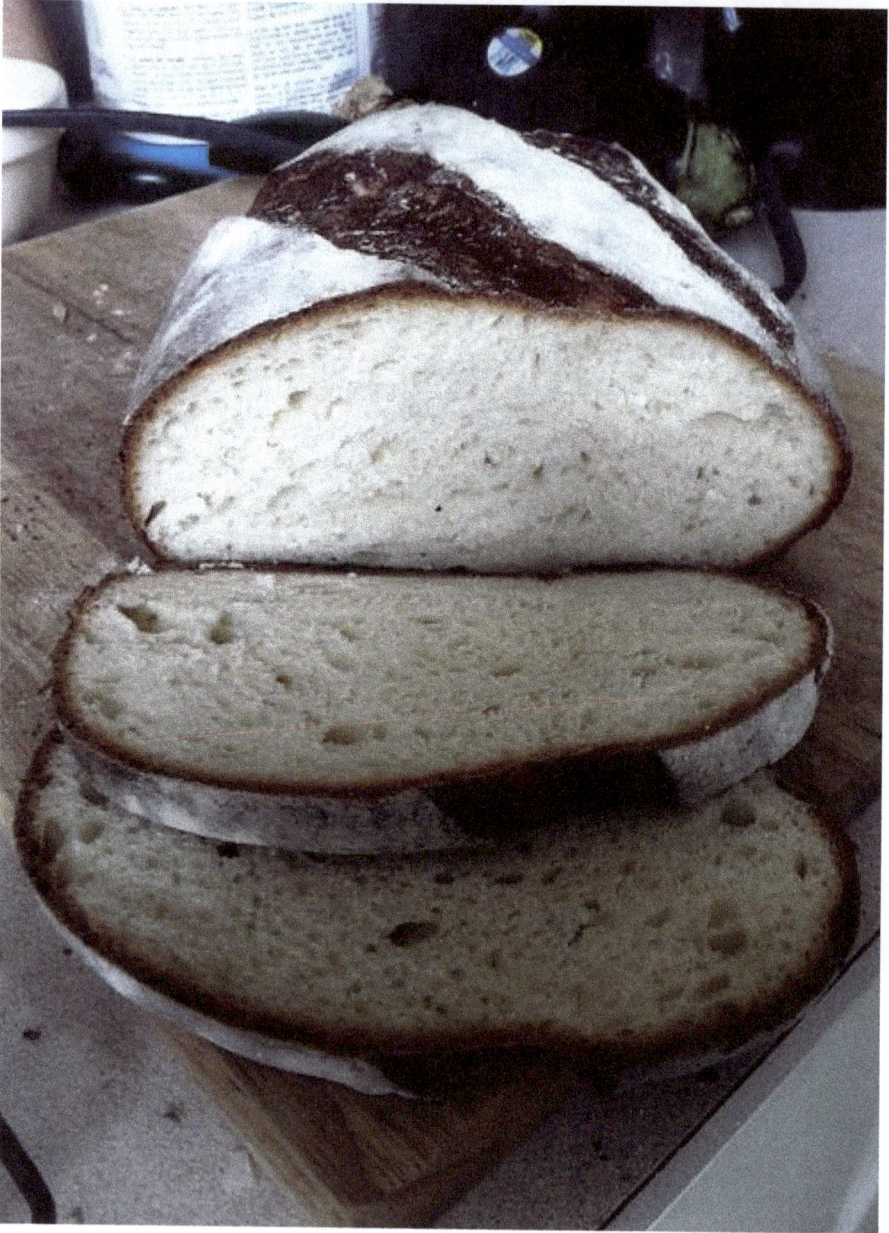

COPYRIGHT

Table of Contents

Country-Style White Bread

Preparation Time: 10 minutes

Ingredients:

1½ cups Lukewarm water

1½ tablespoons Extra-virgin olive oil

1 cup Plain bread flour

2½ cups White all-purpose flour

¼ teaspoon Baking soda

1½ teaspoons Sugar

1 pinch Salt

2½ teaspoons Bread machine yeast

Directions:

1.Add the ingredients into the bread machine as per the order of the ingredients listed above or follow your bread machine's instruction manual.

2.Select the rapid setting and the medium crust function.

3.When ready, turn the bread out onto a drying rack and allow it to cool, then serve.

Tip(s):

1.I made this bread using the rapid cycle on my bread machine. Alternatively, you can make this recipe using the regular setting, adding in only two teaspoons of yeast instead.

2.Check your bread machine when kneading. If the dough appears wet, add in a few teaspoons of flour. If the dough is too thick, put a few teaspoons of water.

Nutrition:

· Calories: 150

· Total fat: 5 g

· Saturated fat: 1 g

· Cholesterol: 0 mg

· Carbohydrates: 17 g

· Dietary fiber: 2 g

· Sodium: 394 mg

· Protein: 2 g

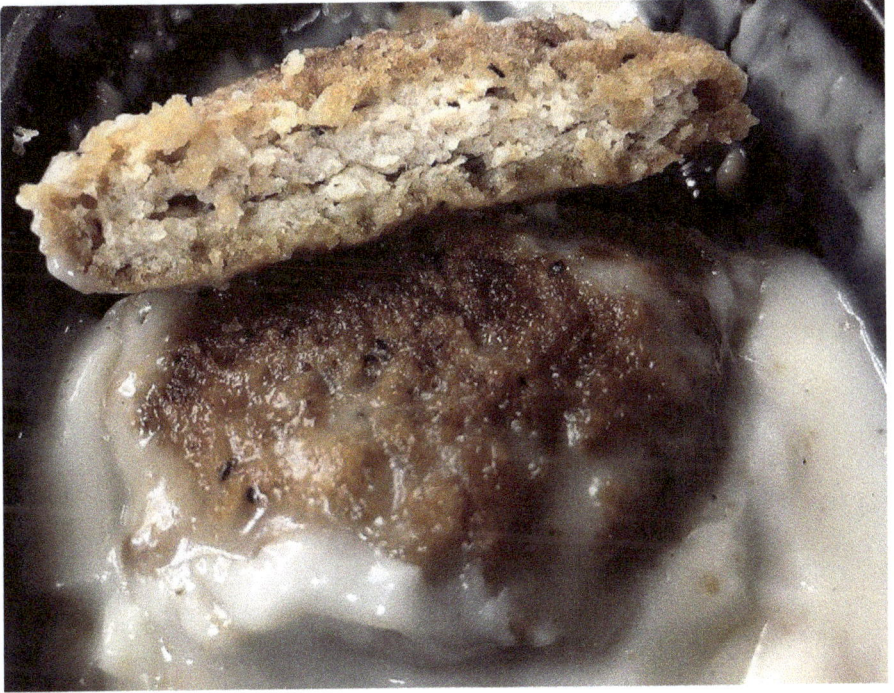

Honey and Milk White Bread

Preparation Time: 5 minutes

Ingredients:

½ cup Lukewarm whole milk

¾ tablespoon Unsalted butter

¾ tablespoon Honey

1½ cups White all-purpose Flour

¾ teaspoon Bread machine yeast

Directions:

1.Add the ingredients into the bread machine as per the order of the ingredients listed above or follow your bread machine's instruction manual.

2.Select the white bread function and the light crust function.

3.When ready, turn the bread out onto a drying rack and allow it to cool, then serve.

Tip(s):

1.You are welcome to add another 1 ½ tablespoons of honey to sweeten the bread further as per your taste.

Nutrition:

· Calories: 162

· Total fat: 1.9 g

· Saturated fat: 0.7 g

· Cholesterol: 2.4 mg

· Carbohydrates: 11 g

· Dietary fiber: 0.7 g

· Sodium: 42 mg

· Protein: 2.9 g

Butter Bread

Preparation Time: 5 minutes

Ingredients:

Egg 1

Lukewarm whole milk 1 cup

Unsalted butter, diced ½ cup

Plain bread flour 2 cups

Salt 1 pinch

Sugar 1 pinch

Instant dry yeast 2 teaspoons

Directions:

1.Add the ingredients into the bread machine as per the order of the ingredients listed above or follow your bread machine's instruction manual.

2.Select the French setting and medium crust function.

3.When ready, turn the bread out onto a drying rack and allow it to cool, then serve.

Tip(s):

1.If your bread maker does not have a French setting, select the white bread function.

Nutrition:

· Calories: 262

· Total fat: 13.5 g

· Saturated fat: 2.2 g

· Cholesterol: 5.6 mg

· Carbohydrates 29 g

· Dietary fiber: 1.3 g

· Sodium: 45.3 mg

· Protein: 5.9 g

Basic White Bread

Preparation Time: 5 minutes

Ingredients:

Lukewarm water ½ cup

Lukewarm whole milk ¼ cup

Unsalted butter, diced 1½ tablespoons

White all-purpose Flour 1¾ cups

Sugar 1½ tablespoon

Salt ¾ teaspoon

Instant dry yeast ¾ teaspoon

Directions:

1.Add the ingredients into the bread machine as per the order of the ingredients listed above or follow your bread machine's instruction manual.

2.Select the basic loaf setting and the medium crust function.

3.When ready, turn the bread out onto a drying rack and allow it to cool, then serve.

Tip(s):

1.This bread can store for up to four days if kept in a cloth bag, away from sunlight.

Nutrition:

· Calories: 160

· Total fat: 2 g

· Saturated fat: 1.3 g

· Cholesterol: 5.5 mg

· Carbohydrates: 1.3 g

· Dietary Fiber: 0.9 g

· Sodium: 130 mg

· Protein: 2.1 ½ g

50/50 Bread

Preparation Time: 5 minutes

Ingredients:

Lukewarm water ½ cup

Honey ½ tablespoon

Unsalted butter, diced 1 tablespoon

Plain bread flour ¾ cup

Whole wheat flour ¾ cup

Brown sugar ¾ tablespoon

Powdered milk ¾ tablespoon

Salt ¾ teaspoon

Instant dry yeast ½ teaspoon

Directions:

1.Add the ingredients into the bread machine as per the order of the ingredients listed above or follow your bread machine's instruction manual.

2.Select the whole-wheat setting and medium crust function.

3.When ready, turn the bread out onto a drying rack and allow it to cool, then serve.

Tip(s):

1.For a less toasted crust, choose the light function on your bread machine.

2.Sprinkle some sesame seeds on top for more flavor.

Nutrition:

· Calories: 166

· Total fat: 2 g

· Saturated fat: 1 g

· Cholesterol: 4 mg

· Carbohydrates: 19 g

· Dietary fiber: 2 g

· Sodium: 235 mg

· Protein: 3 g

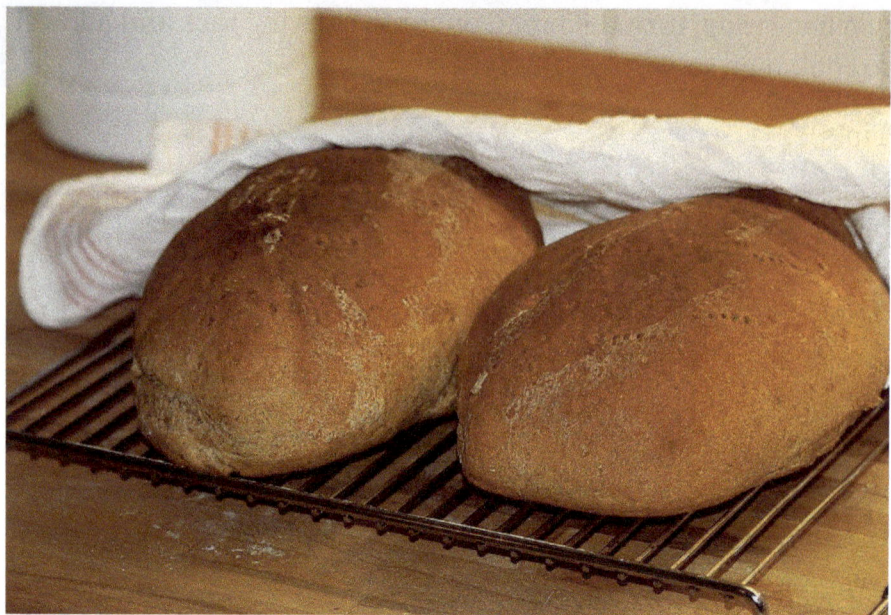

Classic French bread

Preparation Time: 15 minutes

Ingredients:

Lukewarm water 1 cup

Sugar 1 teaspoon

Salt 1 teaspoon

Plain bread flour 3¼ cups

Bread machine yeast 1 teaspoon

Directions:

1.Add the ingredients into the bread machine as per the order of the ingredients listed above or follow your bread machine's instruction manual.

2.Select the French setting and medium crust function.

3.When ready, turn the bread out onto a drying rack and allow it to cool, then serve.

Tip(s):

1.To flavor the bread, add in half a cup of dried cranberries or raisins for a sweeter flavor. For a savory flavor, add in the leaves from two sprigs of rosemary.

Nutrition:

· Calories: 150

· Total Fat: 0.6 g

· Saturated fat: 0.1 g

· Cholesterol: 0 mg

· Carbohydrates: 43.4 g

· Dietary fiber: 1.1 g

· Sodium: 292 mg

· Protein: 5.9 g

Sourdough

Preparation Time: 5 minutes

Ingredients for bread:

Sourdough starter ½ cup

Lukewarm water 1/3 cup

1Sugar ½ tablespoon

Active dry yeast ½ tablespoon

Plain bread flour 1½ cups

Vegetable oil 1½ tablespoons

Salt 1 teaspoon

Ingredients for a sourdough starter:

· 2 cups white, all-purpose flour

· 1 teaspoon active dry yeast

· 2 cups lukewarm water

Directions for a sourdough starter:

1. Add the ingredients in a ceramic or glass dish. Ensure the dish is big enough to allow for expansion.

2. Cover the dish with cloth, fix the cloth into place using an elastic band.

3. Allow the starter to rest for five days in a warm area. Stir the starter once a day.

4. Your starter sourdough is now ready for use. Refrigerate the remainder and use it when needed. If you would like to make a few loaves, you can keep the sourdough starter "alive" by feeding it equal amounts of flour and water and allowing it to rest in a warm area, and using it when needed.

Directions for bread:

1.Add the sourdough starter, water, sugar, and yeast into the bread maker. Using a spatula, combine the ingredients.

2.Allow it to rest for ten minutes.

3.Add bread flour, oil, and salt.

4.Select the basic setting and medium crust function.

5.When ready, turn the bread out onto a drying rack and allow it to cool, then serve.

Nutrition:

· Calories: 180

· Total fat: 4.5 g

· Saturated fat: 0.6 g

· Cholesterol: 0 mg

· Carbohydrates: 30 g

· Dietary fiber: 1.3 g

· Sodium: 467 mg

· Protein: 4.4

French Cheese Bread

Preparation Time: 5 minutes

1½-Pound Loaf

Ingredients:

· 1 teaspoon sugar

· 2¼ teaspoons yeast

· 1¼ cups water

· 3 cups bread flour

· 2 tablespoons parmesan cheese

· 1 teaspoon garlic powder

· 1½ teaspoons salt

Directions:

1.Add each ingredient to the bread machine in the order and at the temperature recommended by your bread machine manufacturer.

2.Close the lid, select the basic bread, medium crust setting on your bread machine, and press start.

3. When the bread machine has finished baking, remove the bread and put it on a cooling rack.

Nutrition:

· Carbohydrates: 21 g

· Fat: 6 g

· Protein: 1½ g

· Calories: 170

· Sodium: 240 mg

Beer Cheese Bread

Preparation Time: 5 minutes

1½-Pound Loaf

Ingredients:

· 1 package active dry yeast

· 3 cups bread flour

· 1 tablespoon sugar

· 1½ teaspoons salt

· 1 tablespoon room temperature butter

· 1¼ cup room temperature beer

· ½ cup shredded or diced American cheese

· ½ cup shredded or diced Monterey jack cheese

Directions:

1.Heat the beer and American cheese in the microwave together until just warm.

2.Add each ingredient to the bread machine in the order and at the temperature recommended by your bread machine manufacturer.

3.Close the lid, select the basic bread, medium crust setting on your bread machine and press start.

4.When the bread machine has finished baking, remove the bread and put it on a cooling rack.

Nutrition:

· Calories: 180

· Carbohydrates: 21 g

· Fat: 5 g

· Protein: 5 g

· Sodium: 360 mg

Jalapeno Cheese Bread

Preparation Time: 5 minutes

1-Pound Loaf

Ingredients:

· 3 cups bread flour

· 1½ teaspoons active dry yeast

· 1 cup water

· 2 tablespoons sugar

· 1 teaspoon salt

· ½ cup shredded cheddar cheese

· ¼ cup diced jalapeno peppers

Directions:

1.Add each ingredient to the bread machine in the order and at the temperature recommended by your bread machine manufacturer.

2.Close the lid, select the basic bread, medium crust setting on your bread machine, and press start.

3.When the bread machine has finished baking, remove the bread and put it on a cooling rack.

Nutrition:

· Calories: 185

· Carbohydrates: 22 g

· Fat: 4 g

· Protein: 7 g

· Calories: 150

· Sodium: 290 mg

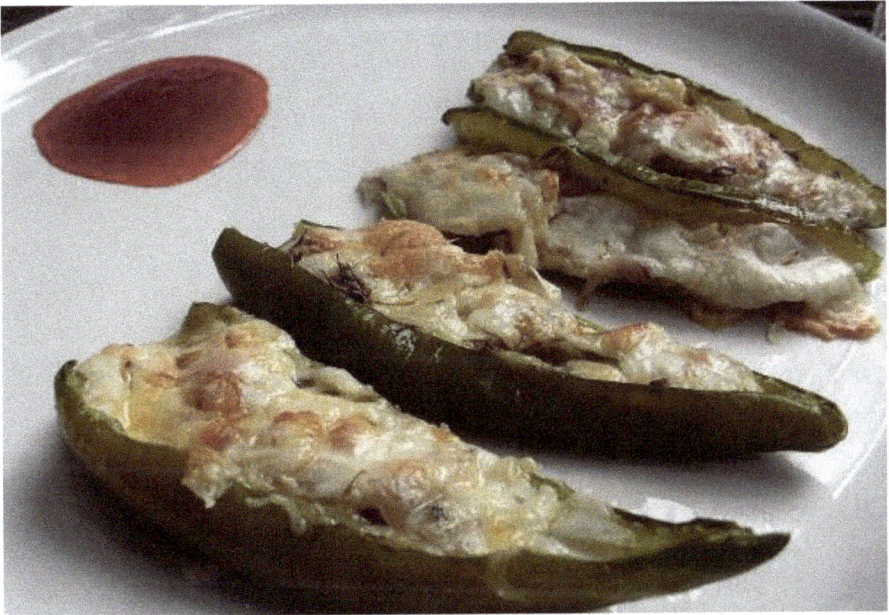

Cheddar Cheese Bread

Preparation Time: 5 minutes

1-Pound Loaf

Ingredients:

· 1 cup lukewarm milk

· 3 cups all-purpose flour

· 1¼ teaspoons salt

· 1 teaspoon tabasco sauce, optional

· ¼ cup Vermont cheese powder

· 1 tablespoon sugar

· 1 cup grated cheddar cheese, firmly packed

· 1½ teaspoons instant yeast

Directions:

1.Add each ingredient to the bread machine in the order and at the temperature recommended by your bread machine manufacturer.

2.Close the lid, select the basic bread, medium crust setting on your bread machine, and press start.

3.When the bread machine has finished baking, remove the bread and put it on a cooling rack.

Nutrition:

· Calories: 182

· Carbohydrates: 25 g

· Fat: 4 g Protein: 7 g

· Sodium: 300mg

Cottage Cheese and Chive Bread

Preparation Time: 5 minutes

3-Pound Loaf

Ingredients:

· 3½ cups water

· 1 cup cottage cheese

· 1 large egg

· 2 tablespoons butter

· 1½ teaspoons salt

· 3¾ cups white bread flour

· 3 tablespoons dried chives

· 2½ tablespoons granulated sugar

· 2¼ teaspoons active dry yeast

Directions:

1.Add each ingredient to the bread machine in the order and at the temperature recommended by your bread machine manufacturer.

2.Close the lid, select the basic bread, medium crust setting on your bread machine, and press start.

3. When the bread machine has finished baking, remove the bread and put it on a cooling rack.

Nutrition:

· Calories: 196

· Carbohydrates: 33 g

· Fat: 4 g Protein: 7 g

· Sodium 320 mg

Ricotta Bread

Preparation Time: 5 minutes

1-Pound Loaf

Ingredients:

· 3 tablespoons skim milk

· ¼ cup water

· 2/3cups ricotta cheese

· 4 teaspoons unsalted butter, softened to room temperature

· 1 large egg

· 2 tablespoons granulated sugar

· ½ teaspoon salt

· 1½ cups bread flour, + more flour, as needed

· 1 teaspoon active dry yeast

Directions:

1.Add each ingredient to the bread machine in the order and at the temperature recommended by your bread machine manufacturer.

2.Close the lid, select the basic bread, medium crust setting on your bread machine, and press start.

3.When the bread machine has finished baking, remove the bread and put it on a cooling rack.

Nutrition:

· Calories: 174

· Carbohydrates: 3 g

· Fat: 1½ g

· Protein: 11 g

· Sodium: 120 mg

Oregano Cheese Bread

Preparation Time: 5 minutes

1-Pound Loaf

Ingredients:

· 3 cups bread flour

· 1 cup water

· ½ cup freshly grated parmesan cheese

· 3 tablespoons sugar

· 1 tablespoon dried leaf oregano

· 1½ tablespoons olive oil

· 1 teaspoon salt

· 2 teaspoons active dry yeast

Directions:

1.Add each ingredient to the bread machine in the order and at the temperature recommended by your bread machine manufacturer.

2. Close the lid, select the basic bread, medium crust setting on your bread machine, and press start.

3.When the bread machine has finished baking, remove the bread and put it on a cooling rack.

Nutrition:

· Calories: 184

· Carbohydrates: 22 g

· Fat: 5 g

· Protein: 3 g

· Sodium: 240 mg

Spinach and Feta Bread

Preparation Time: 5 minutes

1-Pound Loaf

Ingredients:

· 1 cup water

· 2 teaspoons butter

· 3 cups flour

· 1 teaspoon sugar

· 2 teaspoons instant minced onion

· 1 teaspoon salt

· 1¼ teaspoons instant yeast

· 1 cup crumbled feta

· 1 cup chopped fresh spinach leaves

Directions:

1.Add each ingredient except the cheese and spinach to the bread machine in the order and at the temperature recommended by your bread machine manufacturer.

2.Close the lid, select the basic bread, medium crust setting on your bread machine, and press start.

3.When only 5 minutes are left in the last kneading cycle add the spinach and cheese.

4.When the bread machine has finished baking, remove the bread and put it on a cooling rack.

Nutrition:

· Calories: 184

· Carbohydrates: 5g

· Fat: 6 g

· Protein: 6 g

· Sodium: 240 mg

Italian Cheese Bread

Preparation Time: 5 minutes

1½-Pound Loaf

Ingredients:

· 1¼ cup water

· 3 cups bread flour

· ½ shredded pepper jack cheese

· 2 teaspoons Italian seasoning

· 2 tablespoons brown sugar

· 1½ teaspoons salt

· 2 teaspoons active dry yeast

Directions:

1.Add each ingredient to the bread machine in the order and at the temperature recommended by your bread machine manufacturer.

2.Close the lid, select the basic bread, medium crust setting on your bread machine, and press start.

3.When the bread machine has finished baking, remove the bread and put it on a cooling rack.

Nutrition:

· Calories: 180

· Carbohydrates: 1g

· Fat: 6 g

· Protein: 7 g

· Sodium: 350 mg

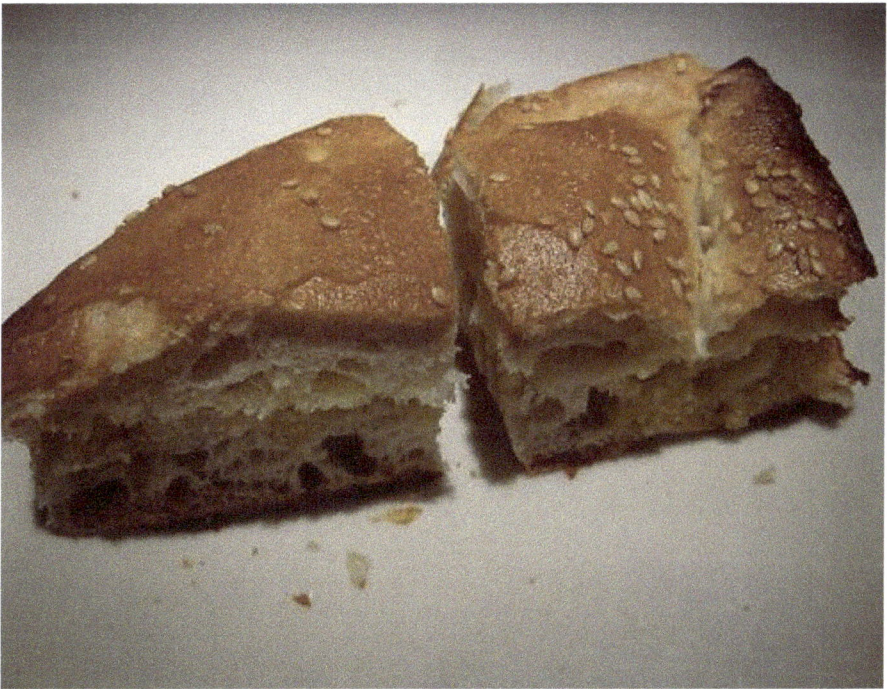

Onion, Garlic, Cheese Bread

Preparation Time: 10 minutes

1½-Pound Loaf

Ingredients:

· 3 tablespoons dried minced onion

· 3 cups bread flour

· 2 teaspoons garlic powder

· 2 teaspoons Active dry yeast

· 2 tablespoons white sugar

· 2 tablespoons margarine

· 2 tablespoons dry milk powder

· 1 cup shredded sharp cheddar cheese

· 1½ cups warm water

· 1½ teaspoons salt

Directions:

1.In the order suggested by the manufacturer, put the flour, water, powdered milk, margarine or butter, salt, and yeast in the bread pan.

2.Press the basic cycle with a light crust. When the manufacturer directs the sound alerts, add two teaspoons of the onion flakes, the garlic powder, and shredded cheese.

3.After the last kneed, sprinkle the remaining onion flakes over the dough.

Nutrition:

· Total Fat: 6 g

· Carbohydrates: 29

· Protein: 12 g

· Sodium: 380 mg

Cream Cheese Bread

Preparation Time: 10 minutes

1 Pound- Loaf

Ingredients:

· ½ cup water

· ½ cup cream cheese, softened

· 2 tablespoons melted butter

· 1 beaten egg

· 4 tablespoons sugar

· 1 teaspoon salt

· 3 cups bread flour

· 1½ teaspoons active dry yeast

Directions:

1.Place the ingredients in the pan in order, as suggested by your bread machine.

2. After removing it from a machine, place it in a greased 9x5 pound pan after the cycle.

3.Cover and let rise until doubled.

4.Bake in a 350° F oven for approximately 35 minutes.

Nutrition:

· Carbohydrates: 24 g

· Total Fat: 5 g

· Protein: 3 g

· Sodium: 240 mg

Mozzarella Cheese and Salami Loaf

Preparation Time: 20 minutes

1-Pound Loaf

Ingredients:

· ¾ cup water

· 1/3 cup mozzarella cheese, shredded

· 4 teaspoons sugar

· 2/3 teaspoon salt

· 2/3 teaspoon dried basil

· Pinch of garlic powder

· 2 cups + 2 tablespoons white bread flour

· 1 teaspoon instant yeast

· ½ cup hot salami, finely diced

Directions:

1.Add the listed ingredients to your bread machine (except salami), following the manufactures instructions.

2.Set the bread machine's program to Basic/White Bread and the crust type to light. Press Start.

3.Let the bread machine work and wait until it beeps. This is your indication to add the remaining ingredients at this point, add the salami.

4.Wait until the remaining bake cycle completes.

5.Once the pound is done, take the bucket out from the bread machine and let it rest for 5 minutes.

6.Gently shake the bucket and remove the pound, transfer the pound to a cooling rack, and slice.

7.Serve and enjoy!

Nutrition:

· Calories: 214

· Carbohydrates: 22 g

· Total Fat: 3 g

· Protein: 6 g

· Sugar: 2 g

· Sodium: 350 mg

Olive and Cheddar Loaf

Preparation Time: 20 minutes

1-Pound Loaf

Ingredients:

· 1 cup water, room temperature

· 4 teaspoons sugar

· ¾ teaspoon salt

· 1 cup sharp cheddar cheese, shredded

· 3 cups bread flour

· 2 teaspoons active dry yeast

· ¾ cup pimiento olives, drained and sliced

Directions:

1. Add the listed ingredients to your bread machine (except salami), following the manufactures instructions.

2. Set the bread machine's program to Basic/White Bread and the crust type to light. Press Start.

3. Let the bread machine work and wait until it beeps. This is your indication to add the remaining ingredients. At this point, add the salami.

4. Wait until the remaining bake cycle completes.

5. Once the pound is done, take the bucket out from the bread machine and let it rest for 5 minutes.

6. Gently shake the bucket and remove the pound, transfer the pound to a cooling rack, and slice.

7. Serve and enjoy!

Nutrition:

· Calories: 190 Carbohydrates: 19 g

· Total Fat: 4 g Protein: 5 g

· Sugar: 5 g Sodium: 300 mg

Cottage Cheese Bread

Preparation Time: 2 hours 50 minutes

Cooking Time: 15 minutes

1-Pound loaf

Ingredients:

· ½ cup water

· 1 cup cottage cheese

· 2 tablespoons margarine

· 1 egg

· 1 tablespoon white sugar

· ¼ teaspoon baking soda

· 1 teaspoon salt

· 3 cups bread flour

· 2 ½ teaspoons active dry yeast

Directions:

1.Into the bread machine, place the ingredients according to the manufacturer's order, then push the start button. In case the dough looks too sticky, feel free to use up to half a cup more bread flour.

2.Gently shake the bucket and remove the pound, transfer the pound to a cooling rack, and slice.

3.Serve and enjoy

Nutrition:

· Calories: 191

· Carbohydrates: 26 g

· Cholesterol: 11mg

· Total Fat: 3.6 g

· Protein: 7.3 g

· Sodium: 384 mg

Green Cheese Bread

Preparation Time: 1 hour

1-Pound Loaf

Ingredients:

· ¾ cup lukewarm water

· 1 tablespoon sugar

· 1 teaspoon kosher salt

· 2 tablespoons green cheese

· 1 cup of wheat bread machine flour

· 5 cups whole-grain flour, finely ground

· 1 teaspoon bread machine yeast

· 1 teaspoon ground paprika

Directions:

1.Place all the dry and liquid ingredients, except paprika, in the pan and follow the instructions for your bread machine.

2.Pay particular attention to measuring the ingredients. Use a measuring cup, measuring spoon, and kitchen scales to do so.

3.Dissolve yeast in warm milk with a saucepan and add in the last turn.

4.Add paprika after the beep or place it in the dispenser of the bread machine.

5.Set the baking program to BASIC and the crust type to DARK.

6.If the dough is too wet, adjust the recipe's amount of flour and liquid.

7.When the program has ended, take the pan out of the bread machine and cool for 5 minutes.

8.Shake the pound out of the pan. If necessary, use a spatula.

9.Wrap the bread with a kitchen towel and set it aside for an hour. Otherwise, you can cool it on a wire rack.

Nutrition:

· Calories: 181

· Carbohydrates: 23.6 g

· Cholesterol: 2 g

· Total Fat: 1 g

· Protein: 4.1 g

· Sodium: 304 mg

· Sugar: 1.6 g

Cheesy Chipotle Bread

Preparation Time: 20 minutes

1-Pound Loaf

Ingredients:

· 2/3cup water, 80°F

· 1½ tablespoons sugar

· 1½ tablespoons powdered skim milk

· ¾ teaspoon salt

· ½ teaspoon chipotle chili powder

· 2 cups white bread flour

· ½ cup (2 ounces) shredded sharp Cheddar cheese

· ¾ teaspoon instant yeast

Directions:

1.Place the ingredients in your machine as recommended on it.

2.Make a program on the machine for basic white Bread, select Light or medium crust, and press Start.

3.When the pound is finished, remove the bucket from the machine.

4.Let the pound cool for 5 minutes.

5.Gently shake the bucket and remove the pound and turn it out onto a rack to cool.

Nutrition:

· Calories: 189

· Carbohydrates: 27 g

· Total Fat: 1 g

· Protein: 6 g

· Sodium: 245 m

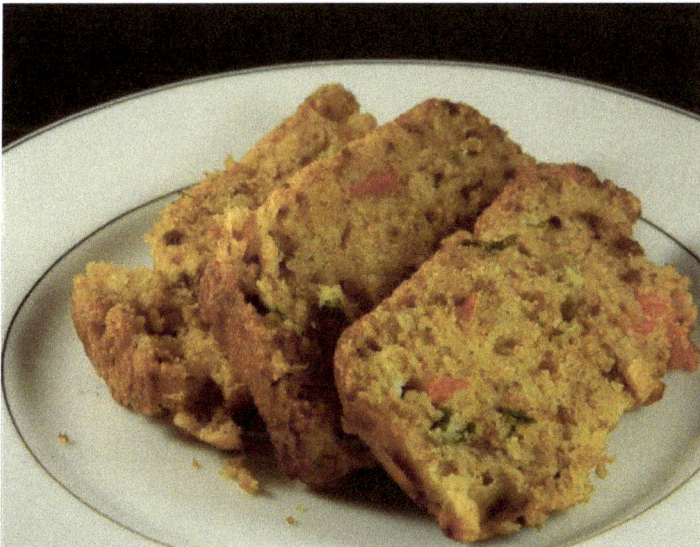

Cheddar Cheese Basil Bread

Preparation Time: 2 hours

1-Pound Loaf

Ingredients:

· 2/3 cup milk, set at 80°F

· 2 teaspoons melted butter, cooled

· 2 teaspoons sugar

· 2/3 teaspoon dried basil

· ½ cup (2 ounces) shredded sharp Cheddar cheese

· ½ teaspoon salt

· 2 cups white bread flour

· 1 teaspoon active dry yeast.

Directions:

1.Place the ingredients in your machine as recommended on it.

2. Make a Program on the machine for basic white Bread, select Light or medium crust, and press Start.

3.When the pound is finished, remove the bucket from the machine.

4.Let the pound cool for 5 minutes.

5.Gently shake the bucket and remove the pound and turn it out onto a rack to cool.

Nutrition:

· Calories: 170

· Carbohydrates: 26 g

· Total Fat: 4 g

· Protein: 6 g

· Sodium: 130 mg

Olive Cheese Bread

Preparation Time: 15 minutes

Ingredients:

· 2/3 cup milk, set at 80°F

· 1 tablespoon melted butter cooled

· 2/3 teaspoon minced garlic

· 1 tablespoon sugar

· 2/3 teaspoon salt

· 2 cups white bread flour

· ½ cup (2 ounces) shredded Swiss cheese

· ¾ teaspoon bread machine or instant yeast

· ¼ cup chopped black olives

Directions:

1.Place the ingredients in your device as recommended on it.

2.Make a program on the machine for basic white Bread, select Light or medium crust, and press Start.

3.When the pound is finished, remove the bucket from the machine.

4.Let the pound cool for 5 minutes.

5.Gently shake the bucket and remove the pound and turn it out onto a rack to cool.

Nutrition:

- · Calories: 175

- · Carbohydrates: 27 g

- · Total Fat: 5 g

- · Protein: 6 g

- · Sodium: 260 mg

Double Cheese Bread

Preparation Time: 2 hours

1-Pound Loaf

Ingredients:

· ¾ cup plus 1 tablespoon milk

· 2 teaspoons butter, melted and cooled

· 4 teaspoons sugar

· 2/3 teaspoon salt

· 1/3 teaspoon freshly ground black pepper

· Pinch cayenne pepper

· 1 cup (4 ounces) shredded aged sharp Cheddar cheese

· 1/3 cup shredded or grated Parmesan cheese

· 2 cups white bread flour

· ¾ teaspoon instant yeast

Directions:

1.Place the ingredients in your machine as recommended on it.

2.Make a program on the machine for Basic White bread, select light or medium crust, and press Start.

3.When the pound is finished, remove the bucket from the machine.

4.Let the pound cool for 5 minutes.

5.Gently shake the bucket and remove the pound and turn it out onto a rack to cool.

Nutrition:

· Calories: 183

· Carbohydrate: 21 g

· Total Fat: 4g

· Protein: 6 g

· Sodium: 244 mg

Chile Cheese Bacon Bread

Preparation Time: 15 minutes

1-Pound Loaf

Ingredients:

· 1/3 cup milk

· 1 teaspoon melted butter cooled

· 1 tablespoon honey

· 1 teaspoon salt

· 1/3 cup chopped and drained green Chile

· 1/3 cup grated Cheddar cheese

· 1/3 cup chopped cooked bacon

· 2 cups white bread flour

· 11/3 teaspoons bread machine or instant yeast

Directions:

1.Place the ingredients in your device as recommended on it.

2.Make a program on the machine for basic white Bread, select Light or medium crust, and press Start.

3.When the pound is finished, remove the bucket from the machine.

4.Let the pound cool for 5 minutes.

5.Gently shake the bucket and remove the pound and turn it out onto a rack to cool.

Nutrition

· Calories: 174

· Carbohydrates: 40 g

· Total Fat: 4 g

· Protein: 6 g

· Sodium: 240 mg

Italian Parmesan Bread

Preparation Time: 5 minutes

1-Pound Loaf

Ingredients:

· ¾ cup water

· 2 tablespoons melted butter

· 2 teaspoons sugar

· 2/3 teaspoon salt

· 11/3 teaspoons chopped fresh basil

· 2 2/3 tablespoons grated Parmesan cheese

· 2 1/3 cups white bread flour

· 1 teaspoon bread machine or instant yeast

Directions:

1.Place the ingredients in your device as recommended on it.

2.Make a program on the machine for Basic White bread, select light or medium crust, and press Start.

3.When it's finished, remove the bucket from the machine.

4.Let the pound cool for 5 minutes.

5.Gently shake the bucket and remove the pound and turn it out onto a rack to cool.

Nutrition:

· Calories: 171

· Carbohydrates: 29 g

· Total Fat: 4 g

· Protein: 5 g

· Sodium: 237 mg

Feta Oregano Bread

Preparation Time: 15 minutes

1-Pound Loaf

Ingredients:

· 2/3 cup of milk, at 80°F

· 2 teaspoons melted butter, cooled

· 2 teaspoons sugar

· 2/3 teaspoon salt

· 2 teaspoons dried oregano

· 2 cups white bread flour

· 1½ teaspoons bread machine or instant yeast

· 2/3 cup (2½ ounces) crumbled feta cheese

Directions:

1.Place the ingredients in your device as recommended on it.

2.Make a program on the machine for Basic White bread, select light or medium crust, and press Start.

3.When it's finished, remove the bucket from the machine.

4.Let the pound cool for 5 minutes.

5.Gently shake the bucket and remove the pound and turn it out onto a rack to cool.

Nutrition:

· Calories: 170

· Carbohydrates: 27 g

· Fat: 4g

· Protein: 5

· Sodium: 180 mg

Awesome Rosemary Bread

Preparation Time: 15 minutes

1 ½-Pound Loaf

Ingredients:

· ¾ cup + 1 tablespoon water

· 12/3 tablespoons melted butter, cooled

· 2 teaspoons sugar

· 1 teaspoon salt

· 1 tablespoon fresh rosemary, chopped

· 2 cups white bread flour

· 11/3 teaspoons instant yeast

Directions:

1.Combine all of the ingredients to your bread machine, carefully following the instructions of the manufacturer.

2.Set the program of your bread machine to Basic/White Bread and set crust type to Medium.

3.Press START.

4.Wait until the cycle completes.

5.Once the pound is ready, take the bucket out and allow the pound to chill for 5 minutes.

6.Gently jiggle the bucket to take out the pound.

Nutrition:

· Carbohydrates: 25g

· Fiber: 1g

· Protein: 4g

· Fat: 3g

· Calories: 1270

· Sodium: 240 mg

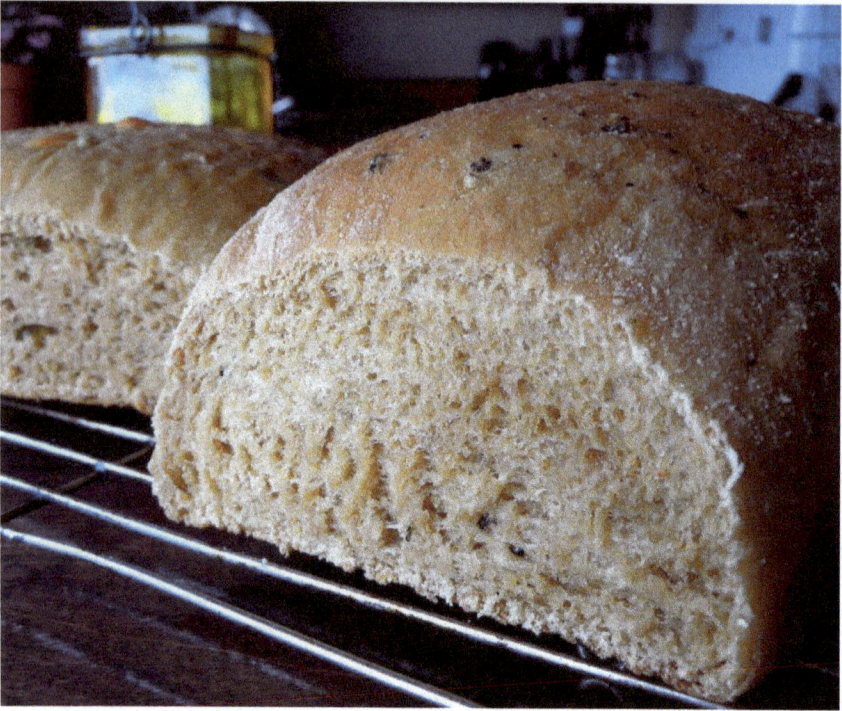

Original Italian Herb Bread

Preparation Time: 15 minutes

1½-Pound Loaf

Ingredients:

· 1 cup water

· ½ cup olive brine

· 1½ tablespoons butter

· 3 tablespoons sugar

· 2 teaspoons salt

· 51/3 cups flour

· 2 teaspoons bread machine yeast

· 1 olive, black/green

· 1½ teaspoons Italian herbs

Directions:

1. Cut olives into pounds.

2. Put all ingredients into your bread machine (except olives), carefully following the instructions of the manufacturer.

3. Set the program of your bread machine to French bread and set crust type to Medium.

4. Once the maker beeps, add olives.

5. Wait until the cycle completes.

6. Once the pound is ready, take the bucket out and cool the pound for 5 minutes.

7. Wobble the bucket to take off the pound.

Nutrition:

· Calories. 180 Carbohydrates: 21 g

· Fiber: 1g Fat: 7g

· Protein: 1g Sodium: 320 mg

Lovely Aromatic Lavender Bread

Preparation Time: 15 minutes

1-Pound Loaf

Ingredients:

· ¾ cup milk

· 1 tablespoon melted butter, cooled

· 1 tablespoon sugar

· ¾ teaspoon salt

· 1 teaspoon fresh lavender flower, chopped

· ¼ teaspoon lemon zest

· ¼ teaspoon fresh thyme, chopped

· 2 cups white bread flour

· ¾ teaspoon instant yeast

Directions:

1.Add all of the ingredients to your bread machine, carefully following the instructions of the manufacturer.

2.Set the program of your bread machine to Basic/White Bread and set crust type to Medium.

3.Wait until the cycle completes.

4.Once the pound is ready, take the bucket out and let the pound cool for 5 minutes.

5.Gently shake the bucket to remove the pound.

Nutrition:

•Calories: 160

•Carbohydrates: 27 g

•Fiber: 1 g

•Protein: 4 g

•Fat: 2 g

•Sodium: 180 mg

Cinnamon & Dried Fruits Bread

Preparation Time: 20 minutes

1-Pound Loaf

Ingredients:

· 2¾ cups flour

· ¾ cup water

· 1½ cups dried fruits

· 4 tablespoons sugar

· 2½ tablespoons butter

· 1 tablespoon milk powder

· 1 teaspoon cinnamon

· ½ teaspoon ground nutmeg

· ¼ teaspoon vanillin

· ½ cup peanuts

· powdered sugar, for sprinkling

· 1 teaspoon salt

· 1½ teaspoon bread machine yeast

Directions:

1.Add all of the ingredients to your bread machine (except peanuts and powdered sugar), carefully following the instructions of the manufacturer.

2.Set the program of your bread machine to Basic/White Bread and set crust type to Medium.

3.Once the bread maker beeps, moisten dough with a bit of water and add peanuts.

4.Wait until the cycle completes.

5.Once the pound is ready, take the bucket out and let the pound cool for 5 minutes.

6.Gently shake the bucket to remove the pound.

7.Sprinkle with powdered sugar.

Nutrition:

· Calories: 315

· Carbohydrates: 65 g

· Fiber: 1 g

· Protein: 5 g

· Fat: 4 g

· Sodium: 240 mg

Herbal Garlic Cream Cheese Delight

Preparation Time: 20 minutes

1-Pound Loaf

Ingredients:

· 1/3 cup water

· 1/3 cup herb and garlic cream cheese mix, at room temp

· 1 whole egg, beaten, at room temp

· 4 teaspoons melted butter, cooled

· 1 tablespoon sugar

· 2/3 teaspoon salt

· 2 cups white bread flour

· 1 teaspoon instant yeast

Directions:

1.Add all of the ingredients to your bread machine, carefully following the instructions of the manufacturer.

2.Set the program of your bread machine to Basic/White Bread and set crust type to Medium.

3.Wait until the cycle completes.

4.Once the pound is ready, take the bucket out and let the pound cool for 5 minutes.

5.Gently shake the bucket to remove the pound.

Nutrition:

· Calories:182

· Carbohydrates: 27 g

· Fiber: 2 g

· Protein: 5 g

· Fat: 6 g

· Sodium: 200 mg

Oregano Mozza-Cheese Bread

Preparation Time: 15 minutes

1 ½ -Pound loaf

Ingredients:

· 1 cup (milk + egg) mixture

· ½ cup mozzarella cheese

· 2¼ cups flour

· ¾ cup whole grain flour

· 2 tablespoons sugar

· 1 teaspoon salt

· 2 teaspoons oregano

· 1½ teaspoons dry yeast

Directions:

1.Add all of the ingredients to your bread machine, carefully following the instructions of the manufacturer.

2.Set the program of your bread machine to Basic/White Bread and set crust type to Dark.

3.Wait until the cycle completes.

4.Once the pound is ready, take the bucket out and let the pound cool for 5 minutes.

5.Gently shake the bucket to remove the pound.

Nutrition:

· Calories: 190

· Carbohydrates: 40 g

· Fiber: 1g

· Protein: 7.7g

· Fat: 2.1g

· Sodium: 220 mg

Cumin Tossed Fancy Bread

Preparation Time: 10 minutes

2-Pound Loaf

Ingredients:

· 5 1/3 cups wheat flour

· 1½ teaspoons salt

· 1½ tablespoons sugar

· 1 tablespoon dry yeast

· 1¾ cups water

· 2 tablespoons cumin

· 3 tablespoons sunflower oil

Directions:

1.Add warm water to the bread machine bucket.

2.Add salt, sugar, and sunflower oil.

3.Sift in wheat flour and add yeast.

4.Set the program of your bread machine to French bread and set crust type to Medium.

5.Once the maker beeps, add cumin.

6.Wait until the cycle completes.

7.Once the pound is ready, take the bucket out and let the pound cool for 5 minutes.

8.Gently shake the bucket to remove the pound.

Nutrition:

· Calories: 161

· Carbohydrates: 67 g

· Fiber: 2g

· Protein: 9.5g

· Fat: 7g

· Sodium: 220 mg

Potato Rosemary Loaf

Preparation Time: 25 minutes

1½ Pound Loaf

Ingredients:

· 4 cups wheat flour

· 1 tablespoon sugar

· 1 tablespoon sunflower oil

· 1½ teaspoons salt

· 1½ cups water

· 1 teaspoon dry yeast

· 1 cup mashed potatoes, ground through a sieve

· crushed rosemary to taste

Directions:

1. Add flour, salt, and sugar to the bread maker bucket and attach mixing paddle.

2. Add sunflower oil and water.

3. Put in yeast as directed.

4. Set the program of your bread machine to Bread with Filling mode and set crust type to Medium.

5. Once the bread maker beeps and signals to add more ingredients, open the lid, add mashed potatoes, and chopped rosemary.

6. Wait until the cycle completes.

7. Once the pound is ready, take the bucket out and let the pound cool for 5 minutes.

8. Gently shake the bucket to remove the pound.

Nutrition:

· Calories: 276

· Carbohydrates: 54 g

· Fiber: 1 g

· Protein: 12 g

· Fat: 3g

· Sodium: 220 mg

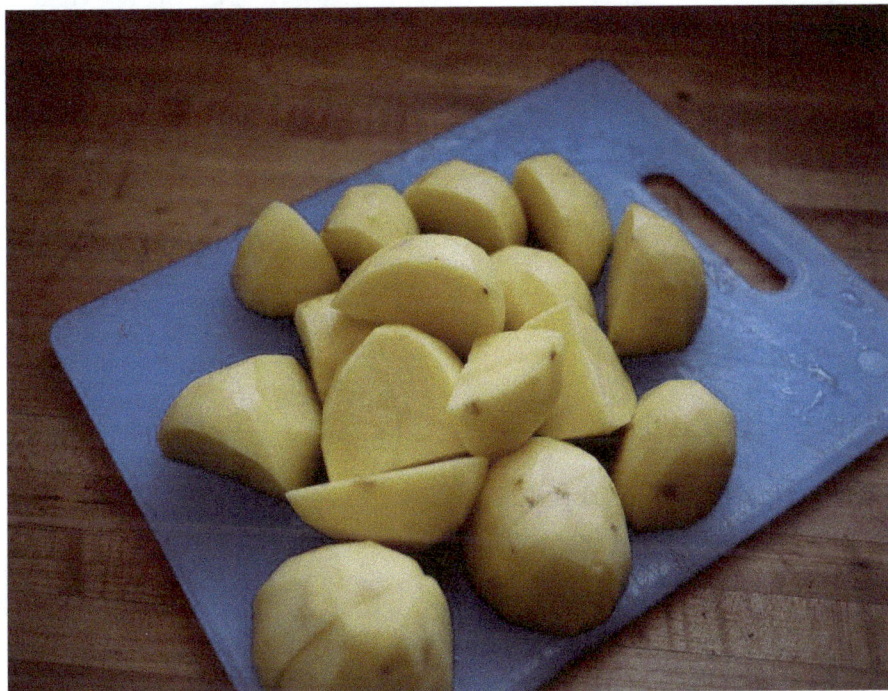

Delicious Honey Lavender Bread

Preparation Time: 20 minutes

1½ Pound Loaf

Ingredients:

· 1½ cups wheat flour

· 21/3 cups whole meal flour

· 1 teaspoon fresh yeast

· 1½ cups water

· 1 teaspoon lavender

· 1½ tablespoons honey

· 1 teaspoon salt

Directions:

1.Sift both types of flour in a bowl and mix.

2.Add all of the ingredients to your bread machine, carefully following the instructions of the manufacturer.

3.Set the program of your bread machine to Basic/White Bread and set crust type to Medium.

4.Wait until the cycle completes.

5.Once the pound is ready, take the bucket out and let the pound cool for 5 minutes.

6.Gently shake the bucket to remove the pound.

Nutrition:

· Calories: 226

· Carbohydrates: 46 g

· Fiber: 1g

· Protein: 7.5g

· Fat: 1.5g

· Sodium: 240 mg

Inspiring Cinnamon Bread

Preparation Time: 15 minutes

1-Pound Loaf

Ingredients:

· 2/3 cup milk

· 1 whole egg, beaten

· 3 tablespoons melted butter, cooled

· 1/3 cup sugar

· 1/3 teaspoon salt

· 1 teaspoon ground cinnamon

· 2 cups white bread flour

· 1 1/3 teaspoons active dry yeast

Directions:

1.Add all of the ingredients to your bread machine, carefully following the instructions of the manufacturer.

2.Set the program of your bread machine to Basic/White Bread and set crust type to Medium.

3.Wait until the cycle completes.

4.Once the pound is ready, take the bucket out and let the pound cool for 5 minutes.

5.Remove the pound

Nutrition:

· Calories: 191

· Carbohydrates: 34 g

· Fiber: 1g

· Protein: 5g

· Fat: 5g

· Sodium: 60 mg

Lavender Buttermilk Bread

Preparation Time: 10 minutes

1½-Pound Loaf

Ingredients:

· ½ cup water

· ½ cup buttermilk

· ¼ cup olive oil

· 3 tablespoons finely chopped fresh lavender leaves

· 1 ¼ teaspoons finely chopped fresh lavender flowers

· grated zest of 1 lemon

· 4 cups bread flour

· 2 teaspoons salt

· 2 ¾ teaspoons bread machine yeast

Directions:

1.Add each ingredient to the bread machine in the order and at the temperature recommended by your bread machine manufacturer.

2.Close the lid, select the basic bread, medium crust setting on your bread machine, and press start.

3.When the bread machine has finished baking, remove the bread and put it on a cooling rack.

Nutrition:

· Calories: 175

· Carbohydrates: 27 g

· Fat: 5 g

· Protein: 2 g

· Calories: 170

· Sodium: 480 mg

Cajun Bread

Preparation Time: 10 minutes

1-Pound Loaf

Ingredients:

· ½ cup water

· ¼ cup chopped onion

· ¼ cup chopped green bell pepper

· 2 teaspoons finely chopped garlic

· 2 teaspoons soft butter

· 2 cups bread flour

· 1 tablespoon sugar

· 1 teaspoon Cajun

· ½ teaspoon salt

· 1 teaspoon active dry yeast

Directions:

1. Add each ingredient to the bread machine in the order and at the temperature recommended by your bread machine manufacturer.

2.Close the lid, select the basic bread, medium crust setting on your bread machine, and press start.

3.When the bread machine has finished baking, remove the bread and put it on a cooling rack.

Nutrition:

· Calories: 170

· Carbohydrates: 23 g

· Fat: 4 g

· Protein: 5 g

· Sodium: 120 mg

Turmeric Bread

Preparation Time: 10 minutes

1 ½-Pound Loaf

Ingredients:

· 1 teaspoon dried yeast

· 4 cups strong white flour

· 1 teaspoon turmeric powder

· 2 teaspoons beetroot powder

· 2 tablespoons olive oil

· 1½ teaspoons salt

· 1 teaspoon chili flakes

· 1½ cups water

Directions:

1.Add each ingredient to the bread machine in the order and at the temperature recommended by your bread machine manufacturer.

2.Close the lid, select the basic bread, medium crust setting on your bread machine, and press start.

3.When the bread machine has finished baking, remove the bread and put it on a cooling rack.

Nutrition:

· Calories: 172

· Carbohydrates: 24 g

· Fat: 3 g

· Protein: 2 g

· Sodium: 360 mg

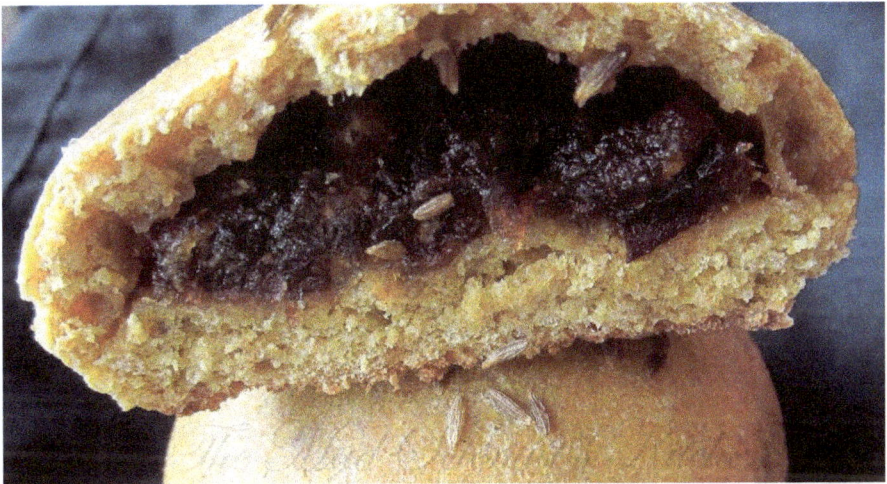

Rosemary Cranberry Pecan Bread

Preparation Time: 10 minutes

2-Pound Loaf

Ingredients:

· 11/3 cups water, plus

· 2 tablespoons water

· 2 tablespoons butter

· 2 teaspoons salt

· 4 cups bread flour

· ¾ cup dried sweetened cranberries

· ¾ cup toasted chopped pecans

· 2 tablespoons non-fat powdered milk

· ¼ cup sugar

· 2 teaspoons yeast

Directions:

1.Add each ingredient to the bread machine in the order and at the temperature recommended by your bread machine manufacturer.

2.Close the lid, select the basic bread, medium crust setting on your bread machine, and press start. When the bread machine has finished baking, remove the bread and put it on a cooling rack.

Nutrition:

· Calories: 171

· Carbohydrates: 12

· Fat: 5

· Protein: 9

· Sodium: 480 mg

Sesame French Bread

Preparation Time: 10 minutes

1½-Pound Loaf

Ingredients:

· 1½ cups water

· 1 tablespoon butter, softened

· 3 cups bread flour

· 2 teaspoons sugar

· 1 teaspoon salt

· 2 teaspoons yeast

· 2 tablespoons sesame seeds toasted

Directions:

1.Add each ingredient to the bread machine in the order and at the temperature recommended by your bread machine manufacturer.

2.Close the lid, select the French bread, medium crust setting on your bread machine, and press start.

3.When the bread machine has finished baking, remove the bread and put it on a cooling rack.

Nutrition:

· Calories: 165

· Carbohydrates: 21

· Fat: 3

· Protein: 6 g

· Sodium: 180 mg

Garlic, Herb, and Cheese Bread

Preparation Time: 20 minutes

1 ½-Pound Loaf

Ingredients:

· ½ cup ghee

· 6 eggs

· 2 cups almond flour

· 1 tablespoon baking powder

· ½ teaspoon Xanthan gum

· 1 cup cheddar cheese, shredded

· 1 tablespoon garlic powder

· 1 tablespoon parsley

· ½ tablespoon oregano

· ½ teaspoon salt

Directions:

1.Lightly beat eggs and ghee before pouring into the bread machine pan.

2.Add the remaining ingredients to the pan.

3.Set bread machine to gluten-free.

4.When the bread is finished, remove the bread pan from the bread machine.

5.Let it cool for a while before transferring it into a cooling rack.

6.You can store your bread for up to 5 days in the refrigerator.

Nutrition:

· Calories: 186

· Carbohydrates: 4 g

· Protein: 5 g

· Fat: 13 g

· Sodium: 120 mg

Savoury Herb Blend Bread

Preparation Time: 20 minutes

1½-Pound Loaf

Ingredients:

· 1 cup almond flour

· 1 cup water

· ½ cup coconut flour

· 1 cup parmesan cheese

· ¾ teaspoon baking powder

· 3 eggs

· 3 tablespoons coconut oil

· ½ tablespoon rosemary

· ½ teaspoon thyme, ground

· ½ teaspoon sage, ground

· ½ teaspoon oregano

· ½ teaspoon garlic powder

· ½ teaspoon onion powder

· ¼ teaspoon salt

Directions:

1.Light beat eggs and coconut oil together before adding to the bread machine pan.

2.Add all the remaining ingredients to the bread machine pan.

3.Set the bread machine to the gluten-free setting.

4.When the bread is finished, remove the bread machine pan from the bread machine.

5.Let cool slightly before transferring to a cooling rack.

6.You can store your bread for up to 7 days.

Nutrition:

· Calories: 180

· Carbohydrates: 6 g

· Protein: 9 g

· Fat: 15 g

· Sodium: 160 mg

Semolina Bread

Preparation Time: 20 minutes

1-Pound Loaf

Ingredients:

· 1 cup almond fine flour

· 1 cup semolina flour

· 1 teaspoon yeast

· 1 egg

· 1 teaspoon salt

· 2 teaspoons Stevia powder

· 2 teaspoons Olive oil extra

· 1 cup warm water

· 2 teaspoons sesame seeds

Directions:

1.Get a mixing container and combine the almond flour, semolina flour, salt, and stevia powder.

2.In another mixing container, combine the egg, extra virgin olive oil, and warm water.

3.By instructions on your machine's manual, pour the ingredients in the bread pan, and follow how to mix in the yeast.

4.Put the bread pan in the machine, select the basic bread setting together with the bread size and crust type, if available, then press start once you have closed the machine's lid.

5.When the bread is ready, open the lid and spread the sesame seeds at the top, and close for a few minutes.

6.By using oven mitts, remove the pan from the machine. Use a stainless spatula to extract the pan's bread and turn the pan upside down on a metallic rack where the bread will cool off before slicing it.

Nutrition:

•Calories: 180

•Carbohydrates: 2.2 g

•Protein: 5g

•Fat: 1g

•Sodium: 200 mg

Seeded Bread

Preparation Time: 10 minutes

1-Pound Loaf

Ingredients:

· 2 tablespoons chia seeds

· ½ cup water

· ¼ teaspoon salt

· 7 large eggs

· ½ easpoon Xanthan gum

· 2 cups almond flour

· 1 teaspoon baking powder

· ½ cup unsalted butter

· 3 tablespoons sesame seeds

· 2 tablespoons olive oil

Directions:

1.Add all the ingredients to the Bread machine.

2.Close the lid and choose Bread mode. Once done, take out from the machine and cut into at least 5 pounds.

3.This seeded bread can be kept for up to 4-5 days in the fridge.

Nutrition:

• Calories: 190

•Fat: 4 g

•Carbohydrates: 4 g

•Protein: 6 g

•Sodium: 150 mg

Macadamia Bread

Preparation Time: 30 minutes

1-Pound loaf

Ingredients:

· ¼ cup almond flour

· ½ cup water

· 1 cup macadamia nuts

· 2 tablespoons flax meal

· 1 teaspoon baking powder

· 2 scoops of whey Protein: powder

· 4 eggs

· 2 egg whites

· 1 tablespoon lemon juice

· ¼ cup butter, melted

Directions:

1.Add all the ingredients to the Bread machine.

Close the lid and choose Express Bake mode. Once done, take out from the machine and cut into at least 5 pounds.

Nutrition:

•Calories: 257

•Fat: 22.4g

• Carbohydrates: 4.5g

•Protein: 11.5g

•Sodium: 20 mg

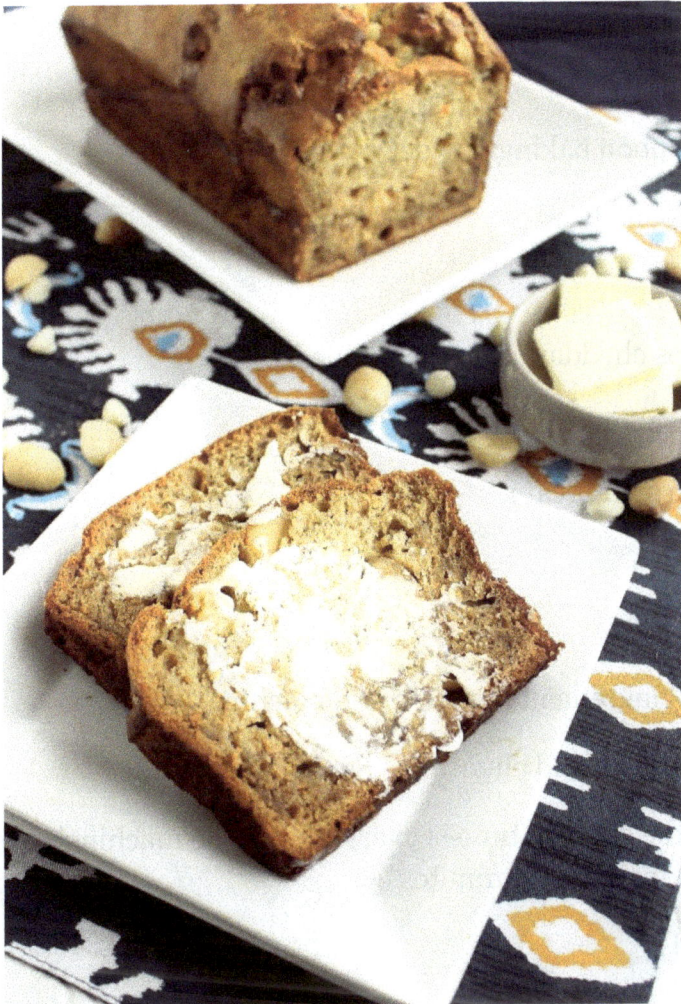

Orangey Almond Bacon Bread

Preparation Time: 10 minutes

1-Pound Loaf

Ingredients:

· 1½ cups almond flour

· ½ cup water

· 1 tablespoon baking powder

· 7 oz bacon, diced

· 2 eggs

· 1½ cups cheddar cheese, shredded

· 4 tablespoons butter, melted

· 1/3 cup sour cream

Directions:

1.Add all ingredients to the bread machine.

2.Close the lid and choose the Sweet Bread mode.

3.After the cooking time is over, remove the machine's bread and rest for about 5 minutes.

4.Enjoy!

Nutrition:

· Calories: 307

· Fat: 26 g

· Carbohydrate: 3 g

· Protein: 1 g

· Sodium: 120 mg

www.ingramcontent.com/pod-product-compliance
Lightning Source LLC
Chambersburg PA
CBHW050750030426
42336CB00012B/1750